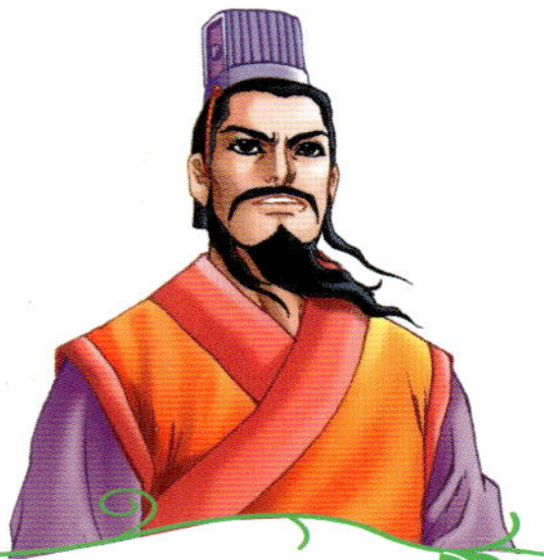

屈原

Qu Yuan

屈原（生於西元前三四零年，逝於西元前二七七年）是戰國時代楚國人。他出身在一個貴族家庭，從小受到良好的教育，加上他不斷的勤奮努力，因此二十多歲便當上楚國的大官。

Qu Yuan was born in 340 BC, and died in 277 BC. He came from an [1]imperial family of the Chu State during [2]Warring States Period. His [3]background and [4]diligence [5]allowed him to become a [6]minister of Chu while he was in his [7]twenties.

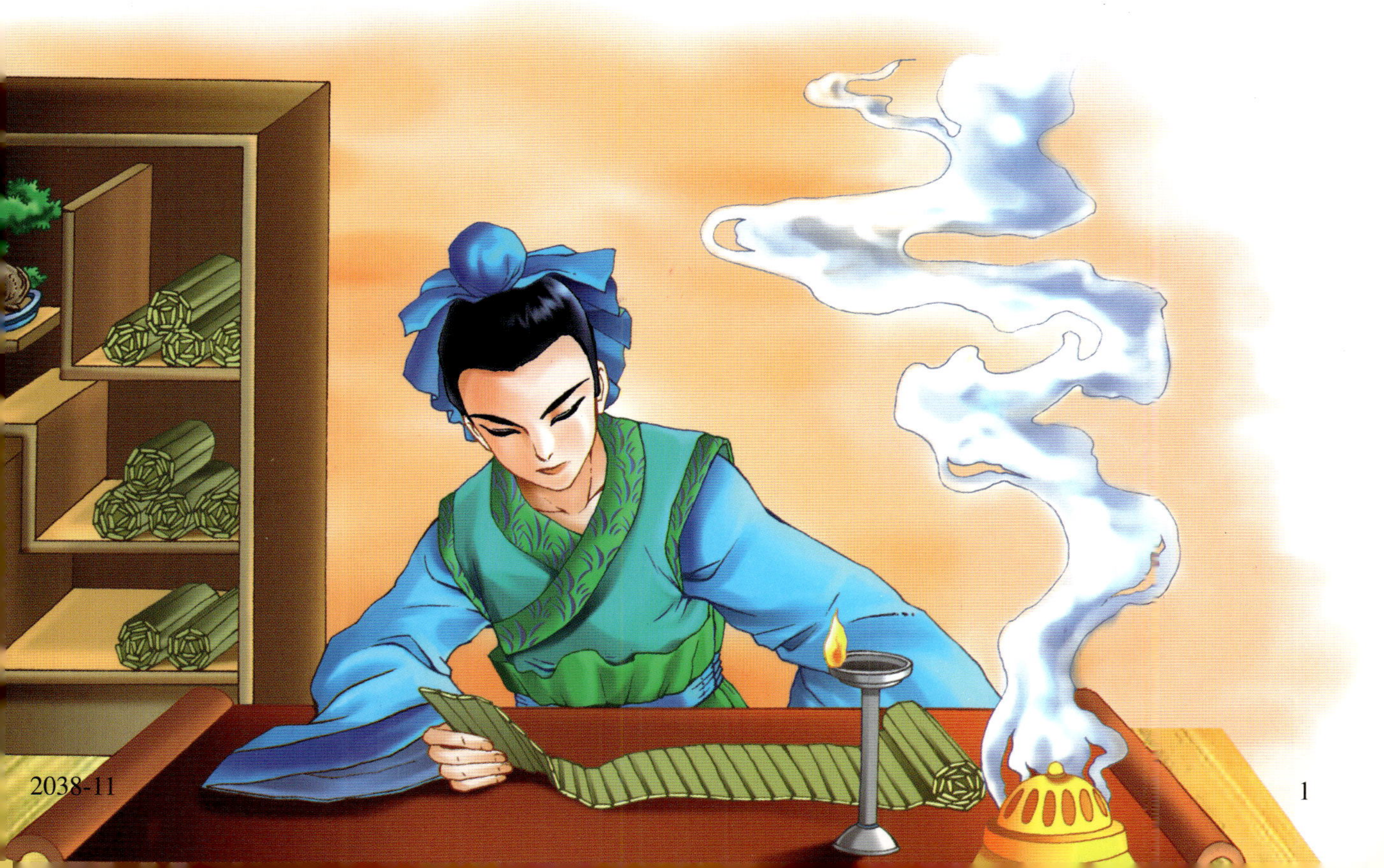

朝廷其他大臣相當嫉妒屈原的才華，經常在楚懷王面前批評他。昏庸的楚懷王，聽信讒言，導致屈原的處境一日不如一日。

當時秦國十分強盛，一心一意要併吞楚國，屈原提出聯合其他國家對抗秦國的策略，但是楚懷王並不接受，最後楚國的軍隊因而節節敗退。

The other ministers at [1] court were very [2] jealous of his talent. They [3] spoke ill of him in front of the King of Chu. Therefore the [4] corrupted king [5] distanced himself from Qu Yuan and took away his [6] position.

Qin was a very [7] powerful state, and was [8] eager to [9] invade Chu. Qu Yuan [10] advocated joining with other states to fight against Qin. The king did not listen. Because of this the [11] troops of Chu was greatly [12] defeated by Qin.

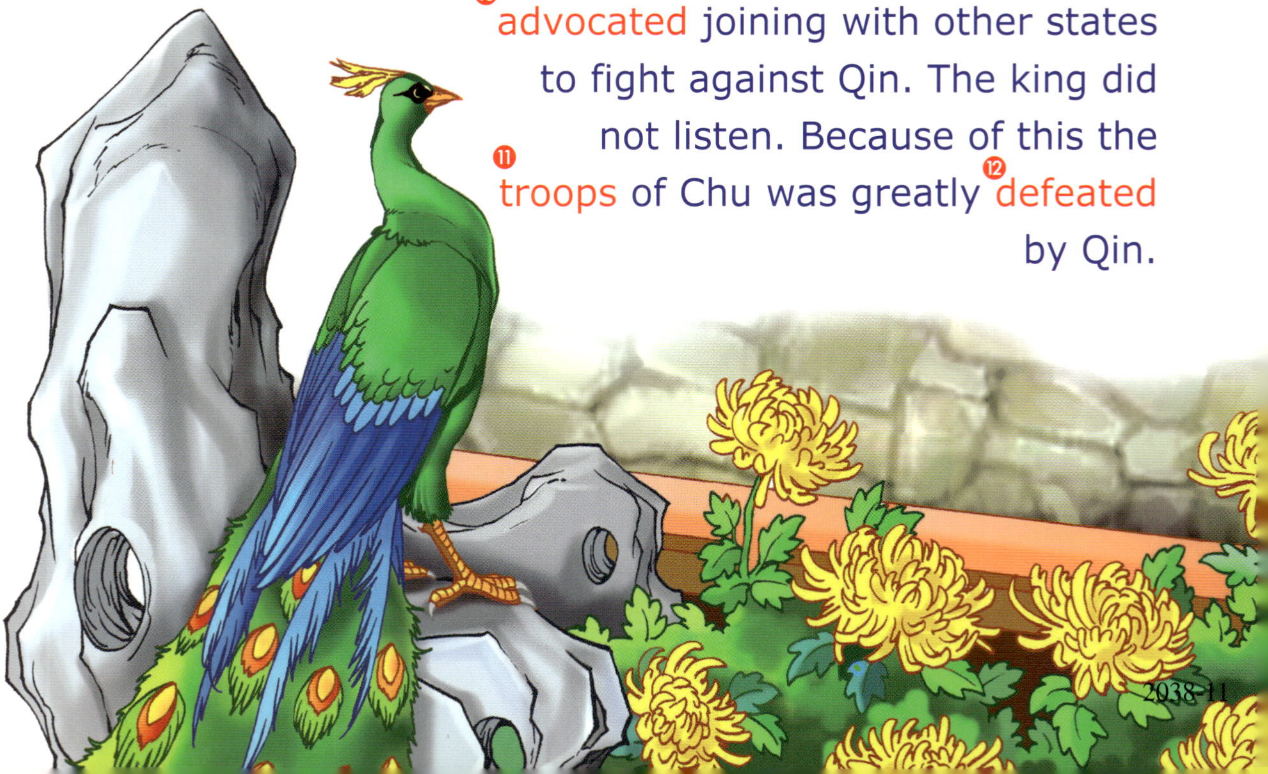

2038-11

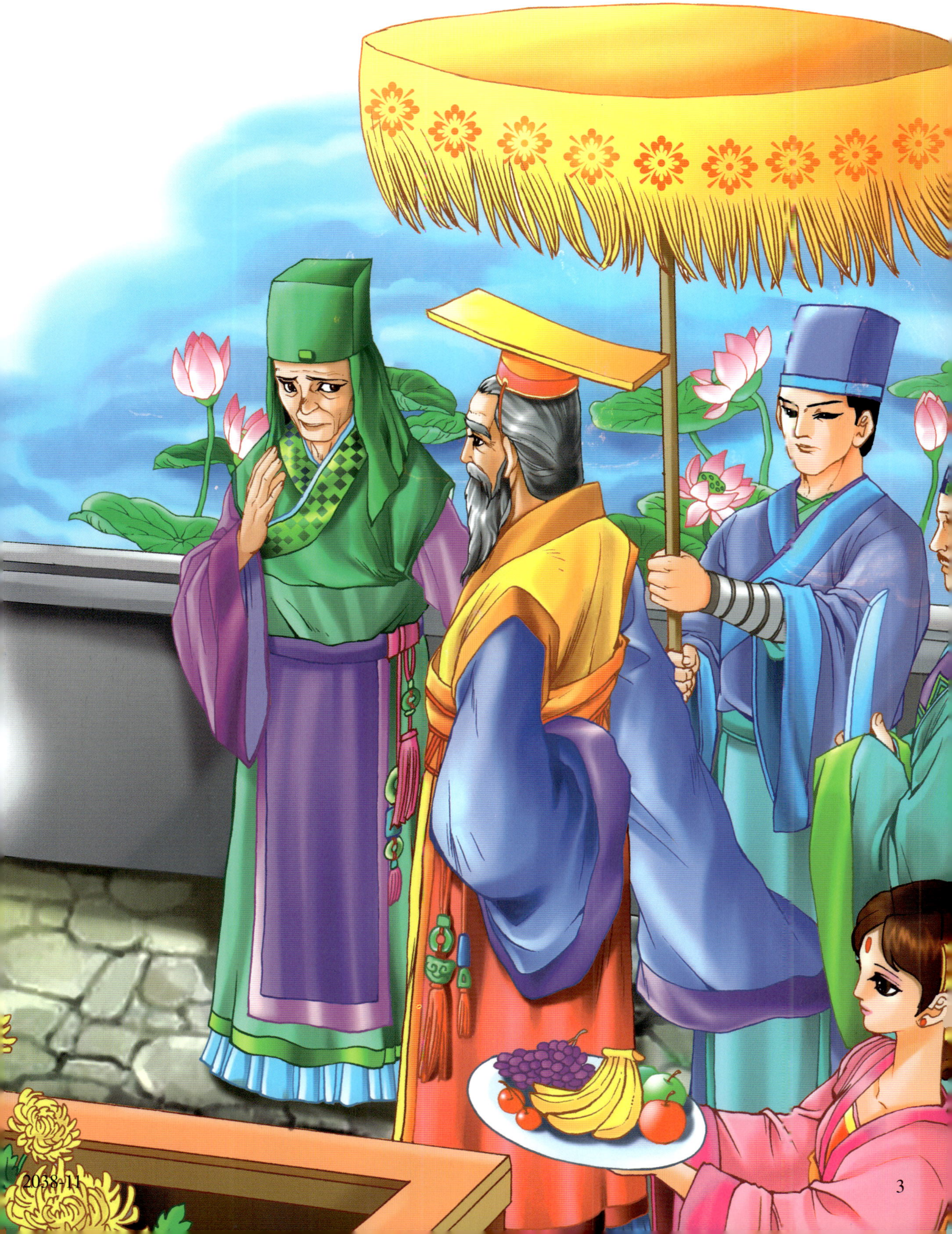

屈原眼見局勢愈來愈差，心中非常著急。在此生死存亡之際，楚懷王還接受秦國之邀，準備到武關共商大事。

屈原看出秦國有詐，然而楚懷王仍然不聽屈原的勸告堅持赴約。後來楚懷王果真在秦國遇害，屈原為此慟哭失聲。

Seeing the ①situation getting worse, Qu Yuan was very ②worried. However, the King of Chu still accepted an ③invitation from Qin to visit.

Qu Yuan ④sensed that something was wrong but the king did not take his ⑤advice. In the end the king was ⑥murdered in Qin. Qu Yuan ⑦wailed ⑧painfully when he heard of the King's death.

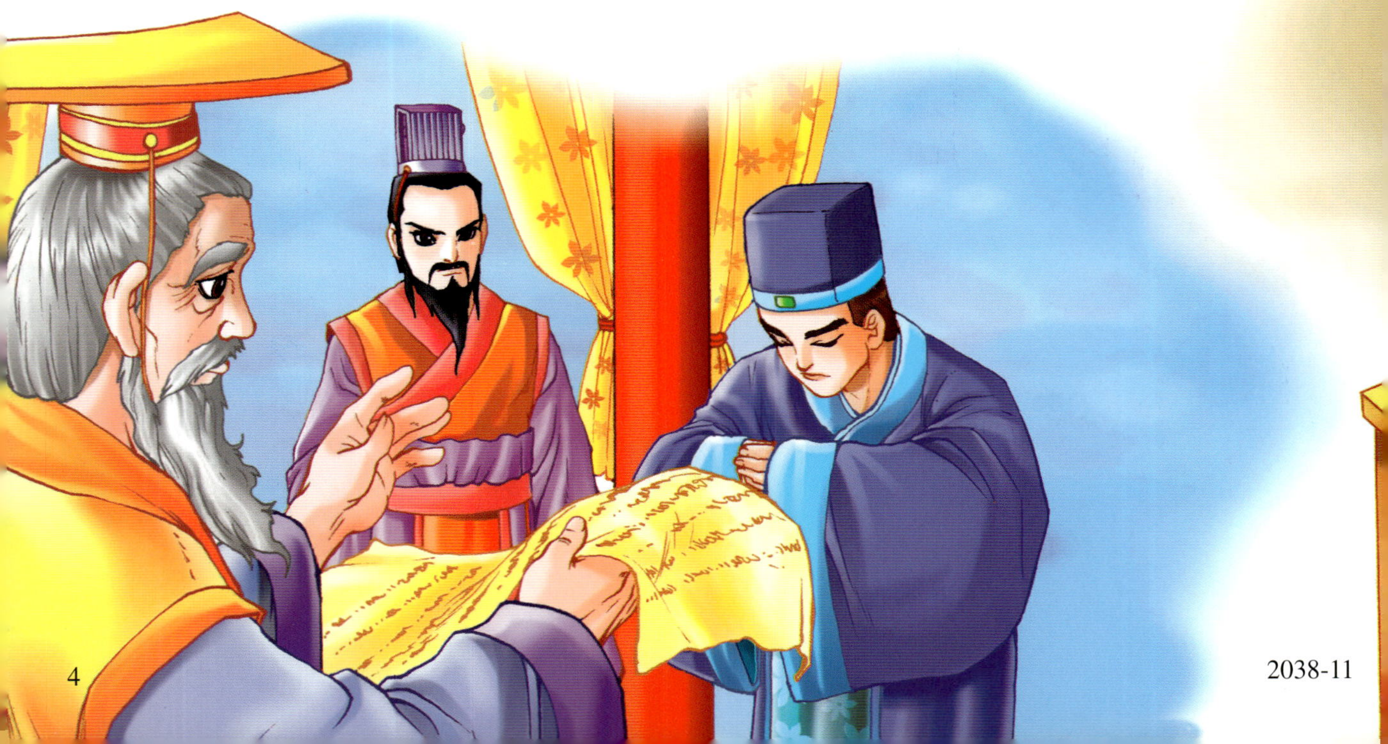

2038-11

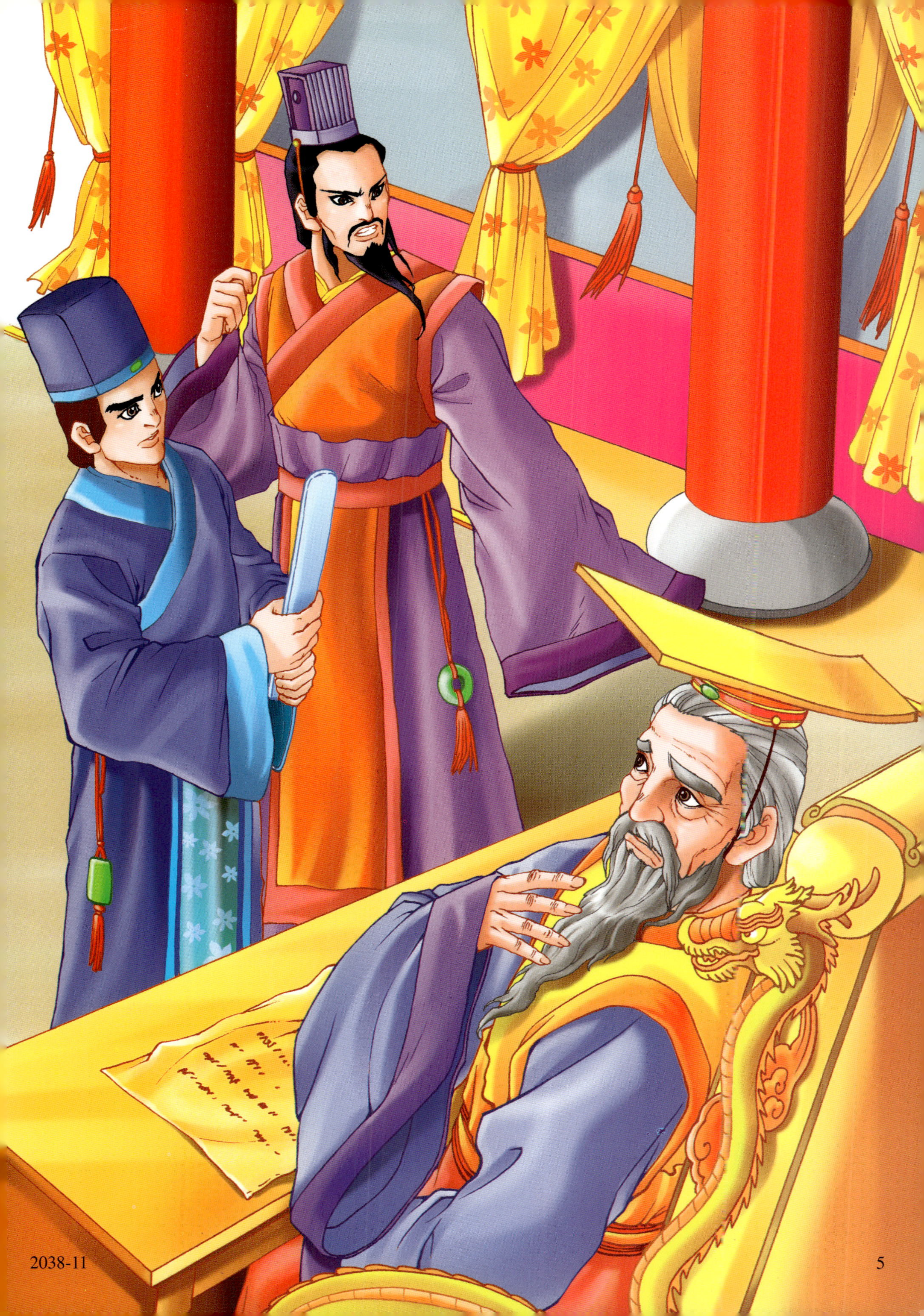

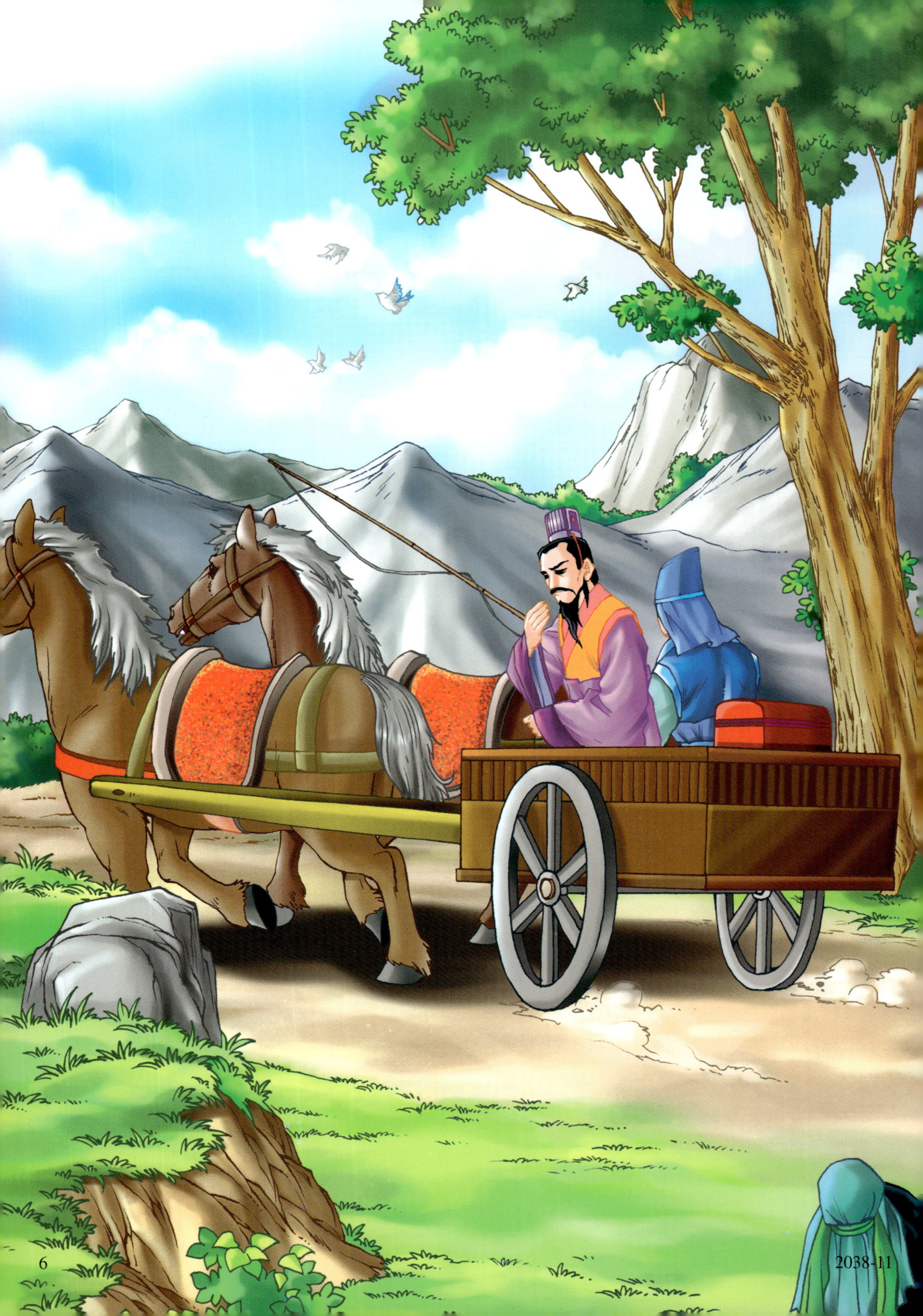

頃襄王繼位後，同樣不肯採用屈原的聯合抗秦政策，甚至還當了秦王的女婿。錯誤的決定讓楚國長期受到屈辱。

屈原內心難過，忍不住寫了批評朝政的詩篇，暗喻大好河山從此蒙羞。頃襄王惱羞成怒，就把屈原流放到南方荒涼之地。

When the new king of Chu came to power, he still ❶ignored Qu Yuan's ❷strategy and even married the King of Qin's daughter. This, along with other wrong decisions put Chu in ❸disgrace.

Not being able to ❹bear his ❺disappointment, Qu Yuan wrote ❻verses that ❼criticized the court, and ❽suggested the disgrace. The king was so ❾furious that he ❿exiled Qu Yuan to the South.

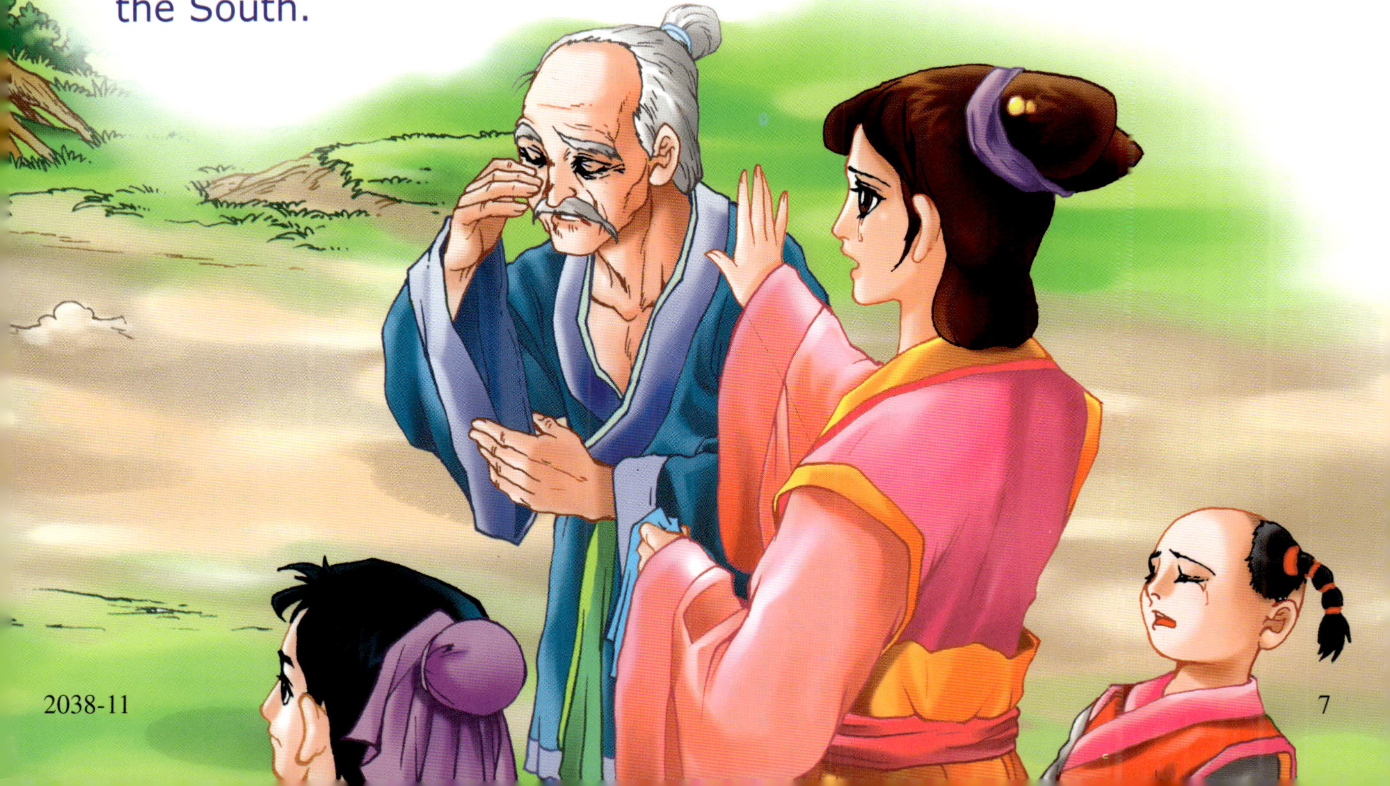

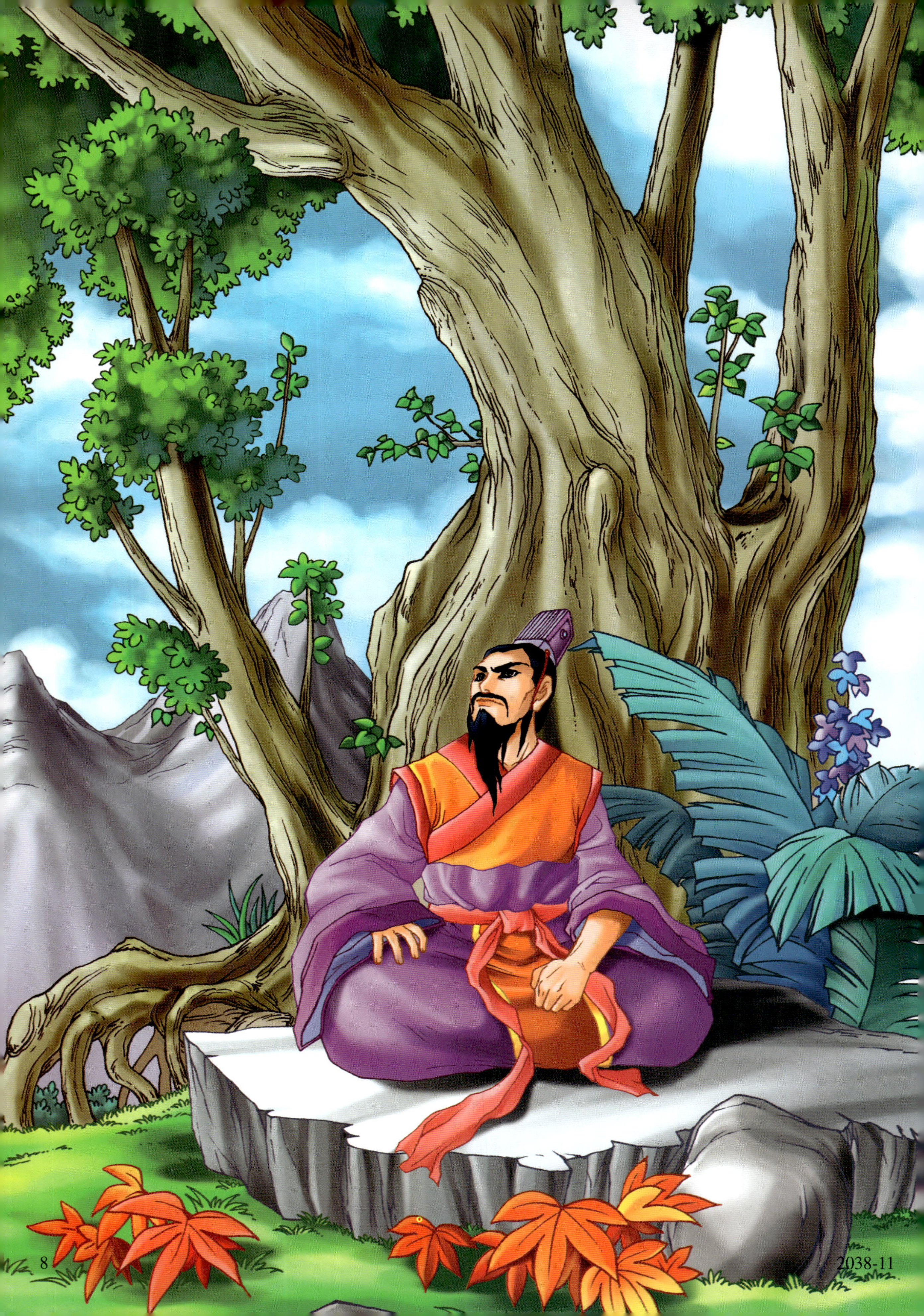

流放的生活十分困苦，屈原常常在深山或江邊苦思，吟誦著自己有感而發所寫的詩篇。

有人看到他生活得如此痛苦，就勸他不要再過問政事，就在南方過著平平淡淡的生活。屈原卻回答說：「國家將亡，人民受苦，我怎能置身事外呢？」

Life during the exile was [1]horrible. Qu Yuan did a lot of thinking while in the [2]countryside and wrote [3]poetry. Some people told him to get away from [4]politics and live a [5]peaceful life in the South. Qu Yuan answered, "How can I be [6]blind to everything, when the country is [7]declining and people are [8]suffering? "

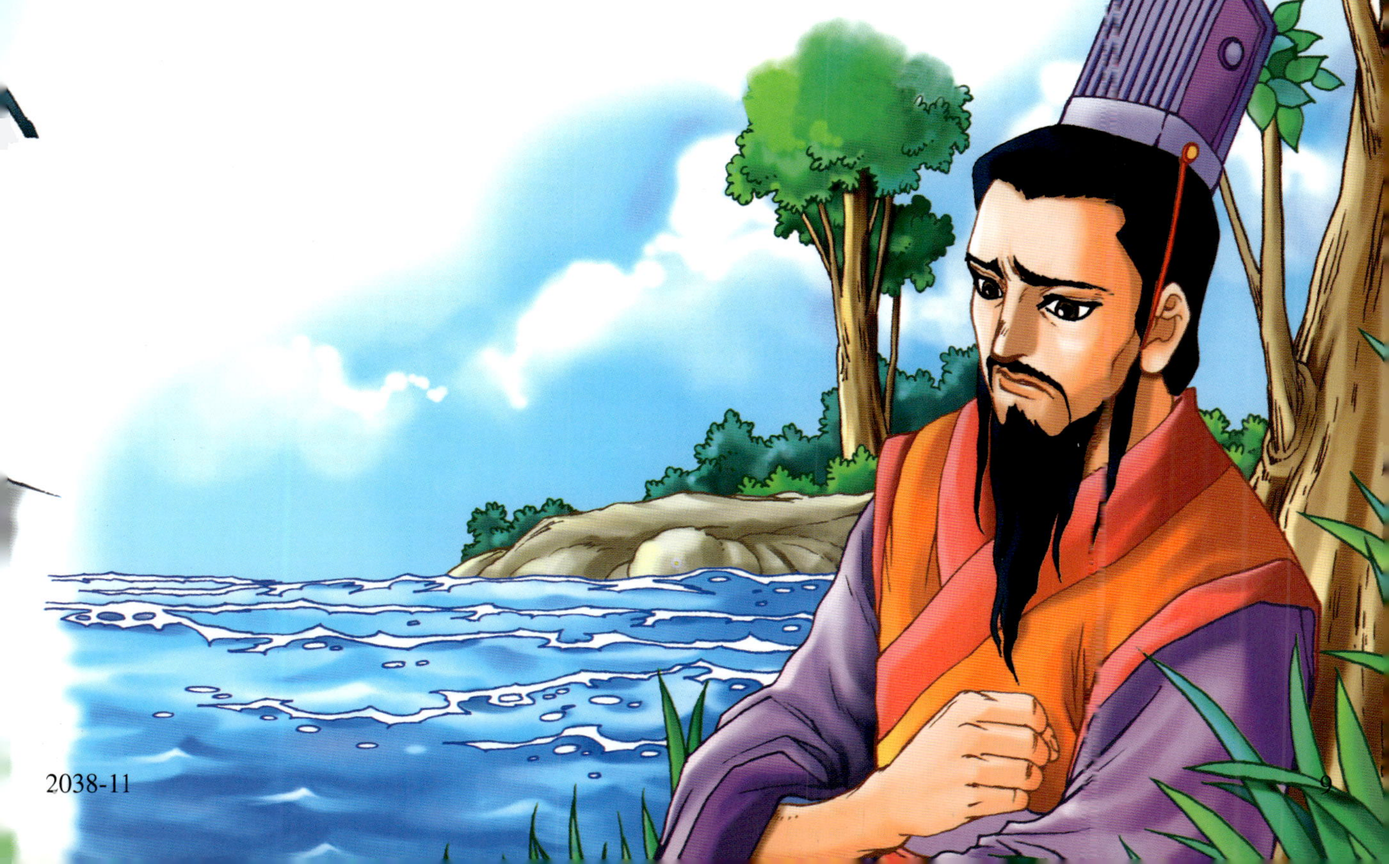

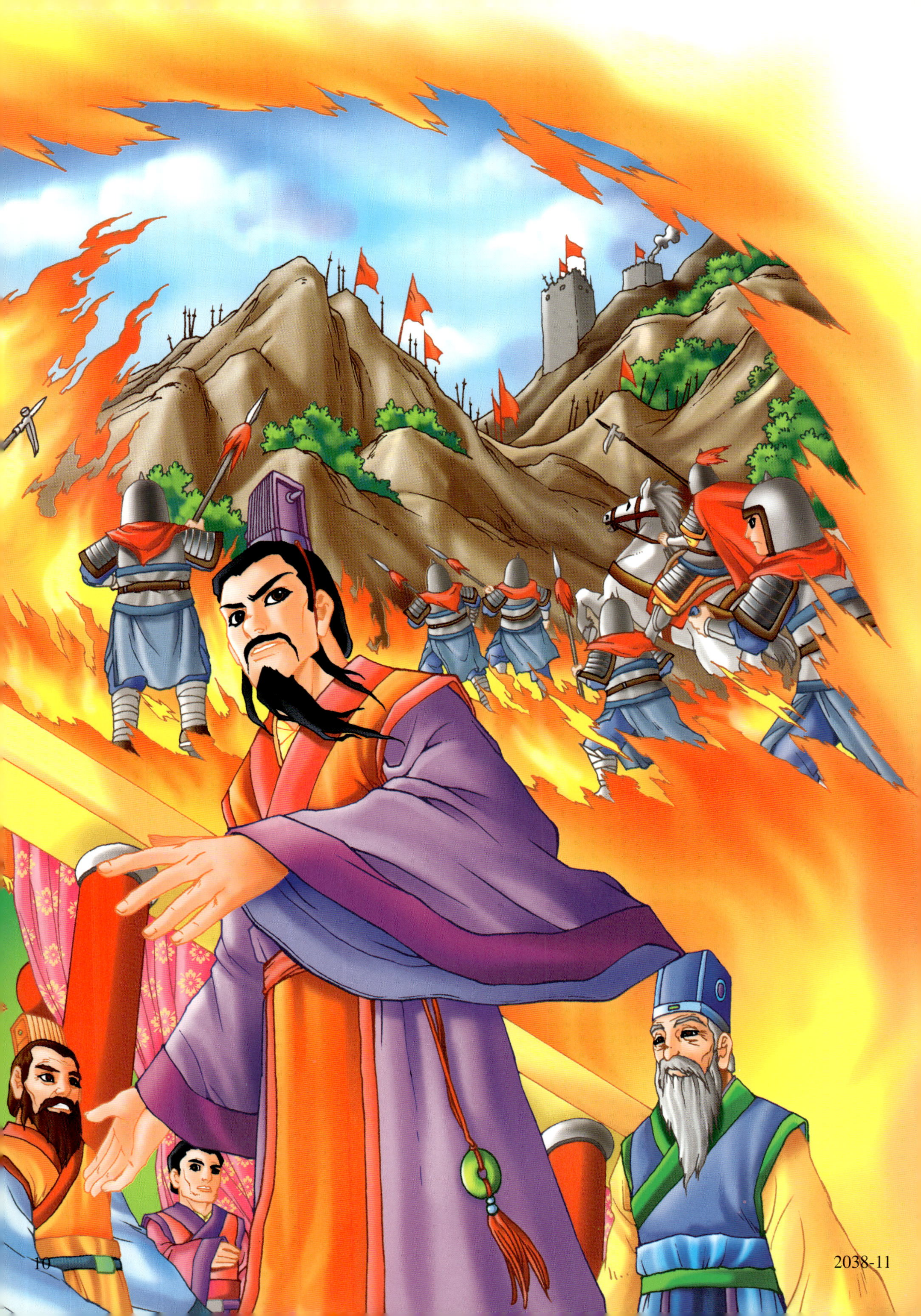

2038-11

　　秦國後來又繼續攻打楚國，楚國陷入困境；屈原趕回京城，想盡辦法要挽救楚國；但是，頃襄王不但拒絕了他的建議，甚至還將他驅逐出境。

　　懷著滿腔愛國熱忱的屈原，無奈於楚王的昏庸，他萬念俱灰的來到汨羅江畔。

Qin [1]launched powerful attacks and [2]weakened Chu. Qu Yuan [3]rushed back to the [4]capital, trying to save his country. But again the king not only [5]rejected his idea, but also ordered him to leave.

Disappointed and [6]upset by the king's [7]corruption, he walked to the [8]riverside of Mi Lo.

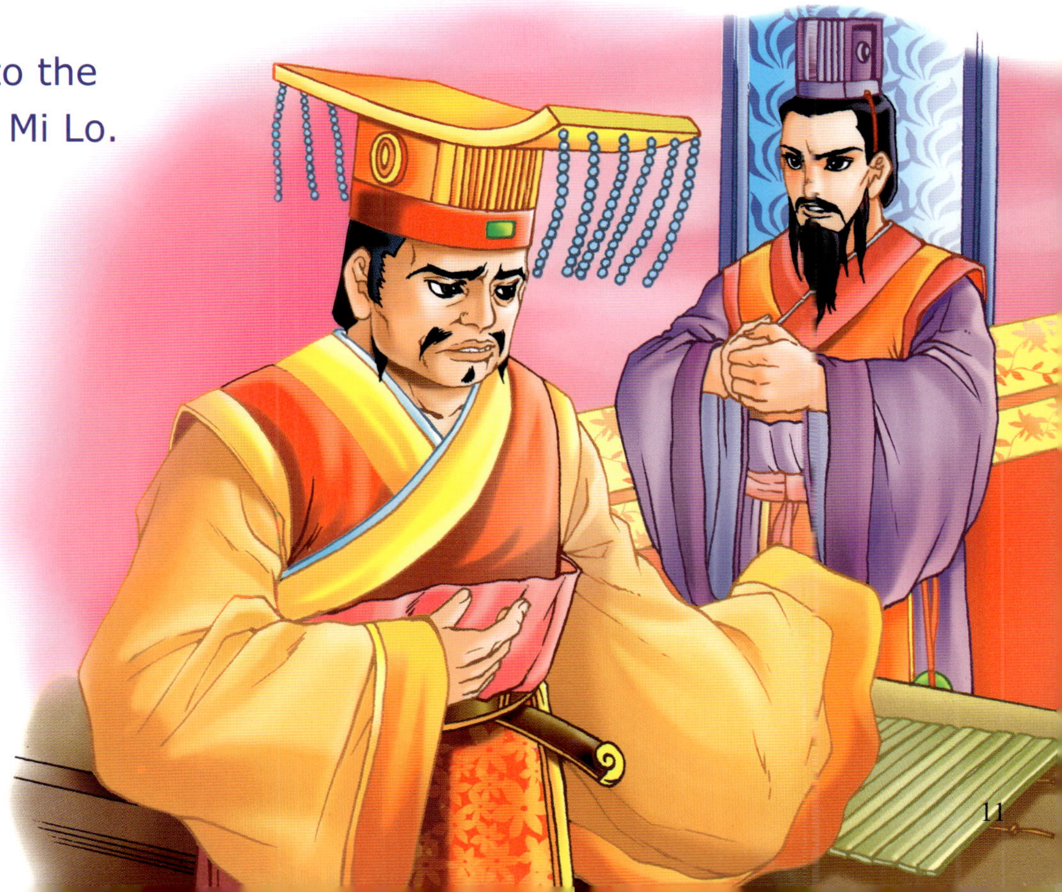

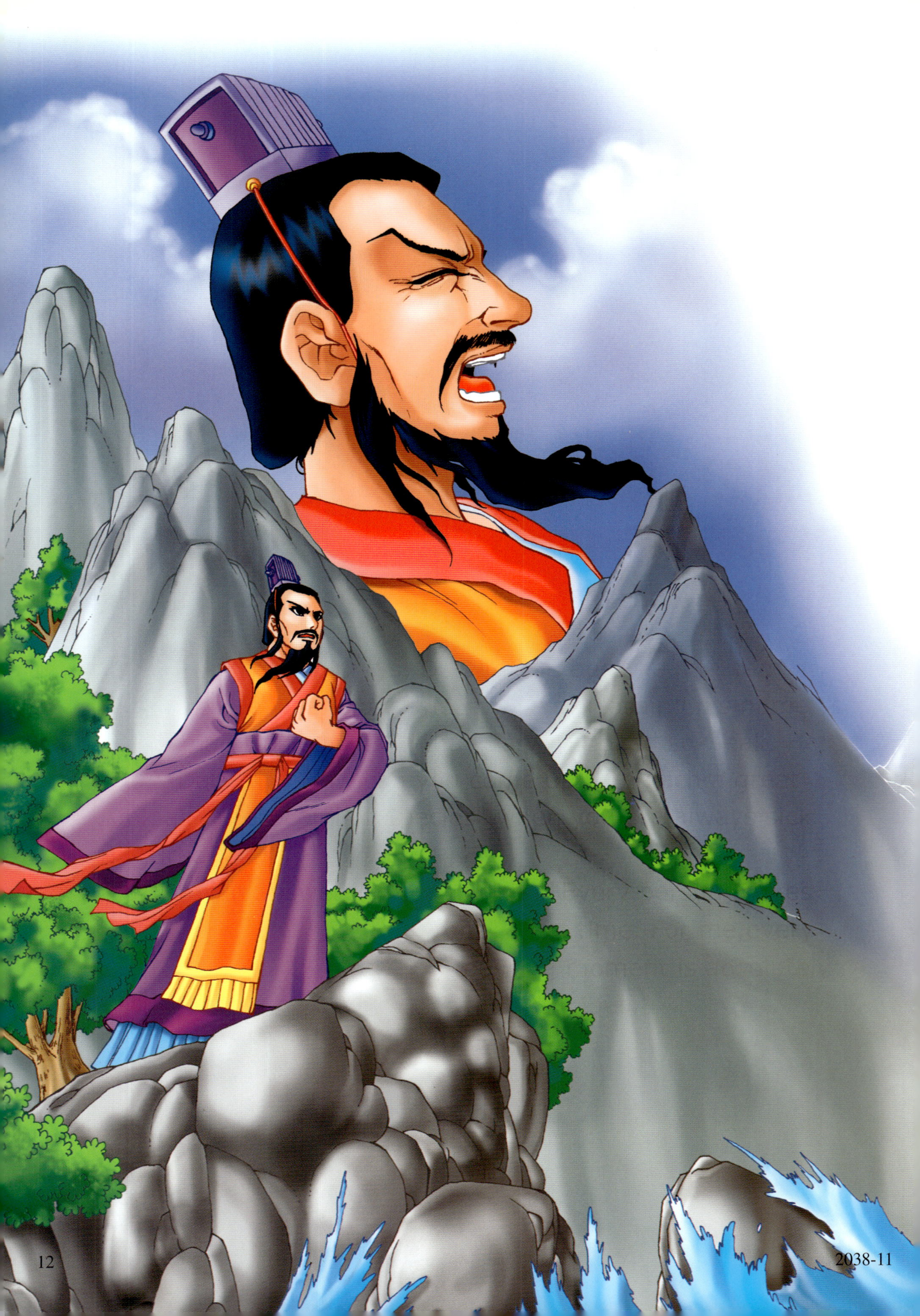

2038-11

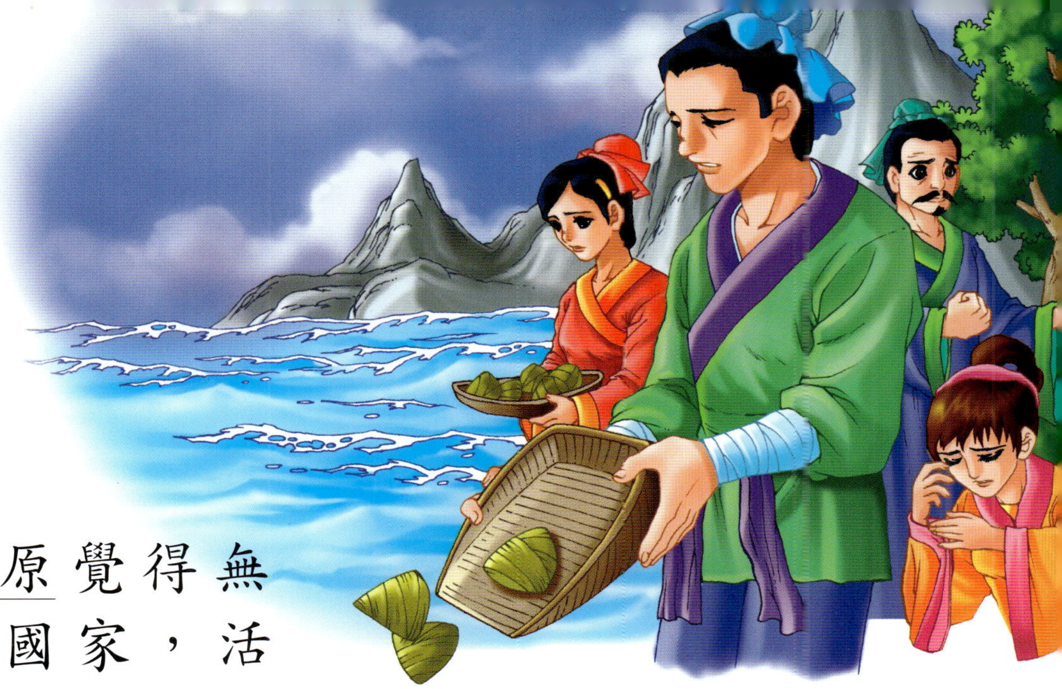

屈原覺得無法報效國家，活在世上已經沒有意義，於是他抱起了大石頭投江自盡，以表達自己對國家的一片忠心。

百姓得知愛國詩人屈原為國捐軀後，紛紛划船趕來搜救，百姓深怕屈原受到江中魚兒的侵食，還特地做了許多粽子丟入江中餵魚，而這也就是農曆五月初五端午節划龍舟、包粽子的由來。

He wasn't able to save his country and thought his life (1) meaningless. So he carried a rock and (2) threw himself into the river to show his (3) loyalty to the king.

People heard about this and (4) raced out on their boats to save him. They threw (5) rice dumplings into the river so that the fish would not eat Qu Yuan's body. Later this became part of the (6) tradition of the (7) Dragon Boat Festival.

讀後心得

屈原一生憂國憂民，滿腔抱負，想拯救日漸衰敗的楚國。他的建議不但沒有被重視，反而處處遭受打壓。最後，只好無奈的投江自盡以表明心志。悲壯的胸懷令人感動，但卻不值得效法，因為結束自己的生命並沒有辦法改變既成的事實。

Qu Yuan [1]devoted his life trying to save his country and people. But all his [2]concerns and [3]suggestions were ignored. Finally, he [4]drowned himself to [5]prove his love for his country. His [6]patriotism was [7]inspiring, but we should not follow his example. After all, we can't change anything by ending our own lives.

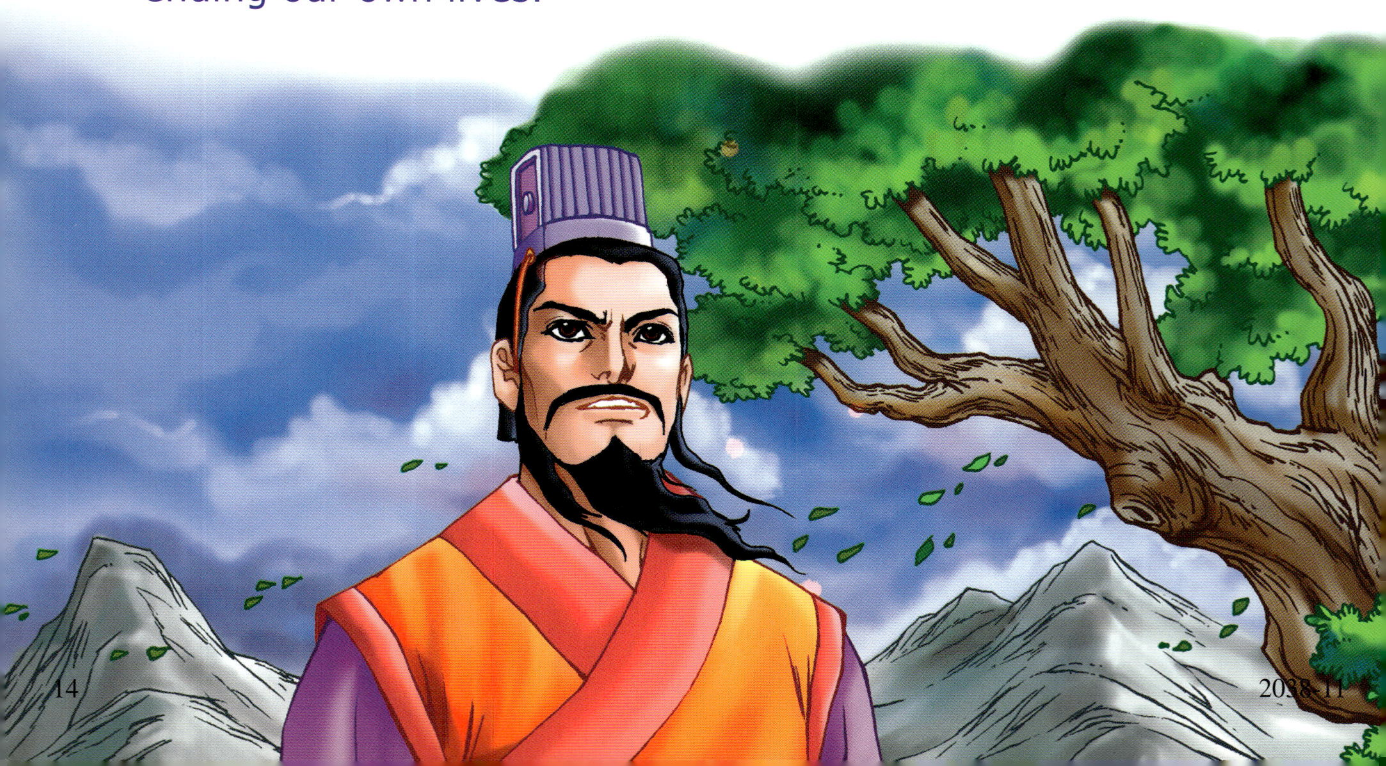

Word Bank

1. imperial 皇家的
2. Warring States Period 戰國時代
3. background 背景
4. diligence 勤勉
5. allow 允許
6. minister 大臣
7. twenties 二十幾歲

P.01

1. court 朝廷
2. jealous 嫉妒的
3. speak ill 說壞話
4. corrupt 腐敗的
5. distance 疏遠
6. position 職位
7. powerful 強大的
8. eager 急切的
9. invade 入侵
10. advocate 提倡
11. troop 軍隊
12. defeat 戰勝

P.02

1. situation 情況
2. worried 擔心的
3. invitation 邀請
4. sense 察覺到
5. advice 建議
6. murder 謀殺
7. wail 慟哭
8. painfully 痛苦的

P.04

1. ignore 忽視
2. strategy 策略
3. disgrace 恥辱
4. bear 承擔
5. disappointment 失望
6. verse 詩篇
7. criticize 批評
8. suggest 暗示
9. furious 憤怒
10. exile 放逐

P.07

Word Bank

1. horrible 可怕的
2. countryside 鄉間
3. poetry 詩
4. politics 政治
5. peaceful 和平的
6. blind 視而不見的
7. decline 衰落
8. suffer 受苦

P.09

1. launch 發動
2. weaken 削弱
3. rush 趕去
4. capital 首都
5. reject 不接受
6. upset 沮喪
7. corruption 腐敗
8. riverside 河邊

P.11

1. meaningless 無意義的
2. throw 把…投進
3. loyalty 忠心
4. race 全速行進
5. rice dumpling 粽子
6. tradition 傳統
7. Dragon Boat Festival 端午節

P.13

1. devote 奉獻
2. concern 憂慮
3. suggestion 建言
4. drown 淹死
5. prove 證明
6. patriotism 愛國心
7. inspiring 令人鼓舞的

P.14